A Parenting Press Qwik Book

What to Do About Sleep Problems in Young Children,

12 Months to 5 Years

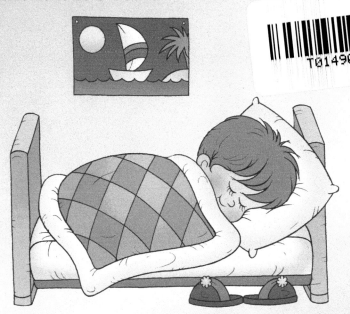

Helen F. Neville, B.S., R.N.

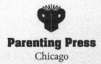

Parenting Press
Chicago

Printed in the United States of America
Designed by Judy Petry

PARENTING PRESS
814 North Franklin Street
Chicago, Illinois 60610
ISBN 978-1-884734-88-5

Contents

Introduction

There is no single right way for families to sleep. Sleep is affected by individual biology, stage of development, family preference, and culture. This book addresses the many reasons parents call for help—night waking, sleep schedules, bedtime resistance, and more.

As a pediatric advice nurse and specialist in inborn temperament, I've been helping families with sleep issues for more than 30 years. Children's sleep is a central issue because it impacts the whole family. None of us do as well when we are short of sleep. Here you will find practical strategies to diminish conflict and restore sleep in your home.

CHAPTER 1: Hope for Tired Parents

Emma refuses to go to bed at night. When left in her room, she screams.

Jesse cries two to four times each night. In a family bed together, his parents didn't expect such difficulties.

Terrell wakes every night with frightening nightmares. Mom calms him but then she can't get back to sleep.

Byron kicks and thrashes next to Mom in their small studio apartment. She hasn't slept well for months.

Beatriz naps at childcare but not at home on the weekends.

Kids are fussy, easily frustrated, and accident prone when short on sleep. Sleep deprivation may also cause headaches and stomach-aches. However, it's more often *parents* who are short of sleep—too exhausted to figure out how to make things better.

If this describes your family, consider ways to catch some extra sleep even temporarily. You'll then have more judgment, creativity, and energy to come up with a longer term plan. Think of it as putting a gallon of gas in an empty tank so you can get to the gas station.

Options for parents to catch up on some sleep:
- **Nap** while the child naps.
- **Share night shifts** with your partner according to what works better for each of you.
- **Take an afternoon nap** at a friend's house, while the friend stays with your child.
- **Spend a night or two away** from home while a friend or family member cares for your child.
- **Let the child sleep in your bed** or in your room for a few nights or several weeks—unless this will be a really difficult pattern to change.
- **Sleep in the child's room** for a few nights or several weeks if the child sleeps better that way.

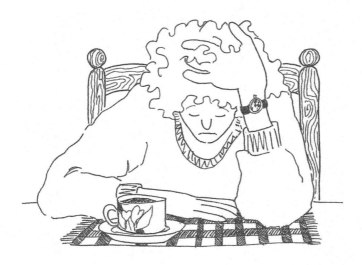

Emma's parents had long morning commutes so they all went to bed at the same time. Now, at 2½, Emma resists bedtime for an hour or more every night. Both parents are exhausted. They decide to "give in" temporarily. Mom takes some sofa pillows into Emma's room and has slept there for two weeks. Emma quickly goes to sleep with Mom in her room. Now that everyone in the family is rested, Emma's parents have the energy to consider next steps.

CHAPTER 2. Keys to Sleep Success

The way to get a good night's rest is to figure out what will work better in *your* family. Sleep needs, inborn temperament, family preferences, and cultures all vary widely. We'll start by looking at what's *not* working in your household. Then we'll look for arrangements that will suit you better.

1. When are you having trouble? Check all that apply, then circle the biggest issue.

○ Getting kids to bed. See p. 10.
○ Getting kids to sleep. See p. 12.
○ Sleep location. See p. 19.
○ Night waking. See p. 21.
○ Naps. See p. 23.
○ Morning issues. See p. 25.
○ Sleep schedules. See p. 27.
○ Nightmares, worry, or stress. See p. 29.

2. Time frame. Is the issue:
New? If yes, has anything changed recently? _____

_____

Ongoing? If yes, why do you want to change now? _____

_____

3. Who is having difficulty?
You? Your partner? The child? A sibling? Others?_____

_____

Are those having trouble a little short of sleep or very short of sleep?

_____

4. How much sleep does your child need? Amounts vary widely among children the same age. Youngsters who wake on their own and are generally in good spirits while awake are usually getting enough sleep. Some children, when overtired, seem wildly energetic and have trouble falling asleep. Because children need less sleep as they grow, they may gradually or suddenly need less sleep. My child generally needs____hours of sleep out of 24.

5. When your child has trouble with sleep, what's going on?
Hungry? In pain? Over-tired or over-stimulated? Lonely? Angry about not getting his/her way? Afraid? Other? _____

_____

6. Ideal versus real goals. Ideally, little ones would look forward to bedtime as much as we do, snuggle for a story, kiss us goodnight, then relax quickly into sleep with that angelic look on their faces. And we'd not hear a peep between 7 P.M. and 7 A.M. What is your goal? Does it seem realistic for your child at this age? _____

_____

_____

Is this a good time to make improvements?
Success is unlikely during illness, travel, or with house guests. Focus on short-term survival at such times. If sleep was disrupted by such factors, it's usually easier to *re*-establish earlier routines again than it was to set them originally. If a new baby is expected, make changes for your toddler or preschooler *beforehand*.

Stages of development affect the ease of making changes. Waiting for a more mellow stage may be well worth it. On the other hand, if you are desperate, or your child has difficulty with changes no matter when they occur, waiting may not be much help.

In terms of general development, easier times for change appear in unshaded sections of this chart.

Why Change Is Easier or Harder	
12-14 mos.	**Easier.** This is well before the "trying 2s." Many toddlers now become attached to a "lovey," which helps them sleep alone.
14 -24 mos.	**More difficult for *some*.** Emotionally intense, strong-minded toddlers enter the "trying 2s" early. Things often get easier around 3.

continued on page 8

7

continued from page 7

2-3 yrs.	**Routines are important.** Two-year-olds don't understand time. To know what's next, they rely on the order of events. Thus routines and rituals help them feel secure and calm.
2½ to 3 yrs.	**More difficulty cooperating.** The natural impulse for independence, control, and personal power makes it hard for these toddlers to do things our way. Their emotions swing widely and resistance is common.
3-4 yrs.	**An easier year.** There's more calm and emotional stability along with better ability to express concerns. Most 3s can sleep easily in a separate room unless frightened by nightmares.
4-5 yrs.	**Less cooperative.** More emotional ups and downs than at 3 and 5 years.
5-6 yrs.	**More flexibility.** A few 5s are somewhat inclined toward worry.

Inborn temperament. Children who are sensitive, emotionally intense, or easily frustrated often have more difficulty with sleep. Some youngsters like new things and adjust easily to transitions and changes while others do not. For the "slow to adapt" children, I prefer to use the term, "natural planner." From a very young age, these kids have a picture in their mind of what they expect to happen next. Many natural planners do better when told ahead of time about changes. Don't avoid important changes just because they are hard for your child. Some moms have endured nighttime breast squeezing or hair tugging for years— afraid to make changes. Resentment can't help but build.

What to work on first? Here are general guidelines.
1. If the child is clearly frightened, handle this first. See p. 29.
2. If the child is hungry at night, change this before other issues. See p. 21.
3. If the sleep schedule isn't working, adjust this next. See p. 27
4. If you need new "sleep cues" (something other than Mom or Dad as the cue for falling asleep), change this *last*. See p. 15.

Mixed feelings about sleep issues? Change is harder when goals conflict. For example, it may be hard to set an early bedtime if your family has been separated all day, yet children may be tired and fussy the next morning if they aren't getting enough sleep. Or, a family bed can be great for family closeness yet may decrease physical intimacy between parents. Consider your priorities. If children sense indecision they will resist change all the more.

Siblings and neighbors. If needed, advise neighbors ahead of time that you'll have several noisy nights. Or, move a sibling to another room for a while. Jesse's older sister slept in the living room for a week while Jesse learned to get back to sleep without nursing at night. (Some youngsters cry less with an older sibling nearby.)

Expect things to get worse before they get better. Changes take extra time and effort on your part. Youngsters often resist or cry. Expect things to be harder for a week or even two.

A Plan to Reach Your Goal

Date _____

Needed change _____

When to start _____
After reading the relevant chapters, list things you can do. Then number which you will do first, second, and third.

_____

_____

_____

What will be hard about this plan? _____

_____

How will you deal with what's hard? Who can help? _____

_____

When do you expect things to be better? _____
    (Expect change in 3-14 days.)
If this plan doesn't work, revise it and try again.

During her first 6 months, Kim screamed every moment she was awake, unless walked or rocked. Now she was a delightful, mellow toddler who nursed briefly once per night. Mom thought Kim would adjust quickly to sleeping through the night, but couldn't bear the thought of her crying. So Mom slept at a neighbor's for two nights. At home, Dad slept through the night, as did Kim upon Mom's return.

Getting children into bed can be a challenge, especially for independent-minded 2s and active 4s. To begin with, start your bedtime ritual after the child is *in bed.* Read stories, give a back rub, or have quiet evening conversation. Looking forward to ritual gives incentive to get into bed.

Here are common issues and things to do:

- **Not tired.** See pp. 6 and 12.
- **Wants more screen time (video or computer or hand-held game) before bed.** Rule: No screen time after dinner (until it's needed for homework).
- **Dawdles while getting ready for bed.** Help kids brush teeth and get dressed if they are less efficient when tired. Ask, "Do you want to walk or be carried to bed?" Set a timer. Kids resent timers less than our nagging. For a timer that even 3s can use get an egg timer or see *www.timetimer.com.* Rule: If you get in bed after the timer rings, story time is shorter or there will be no story.
- **Asks for another story.** Stick to only one or two stories every night. Or set a timer for the number of minutes you will read. If exciting or unfamiliar stories make it hard to stop, read familiar stories at bedtime.
- **Requests one thing after another.** Give two tokens—to exchange for a drink of water, or another hug, or whatever. When tokens are gone, nothing more. Use margarine tub lids, juice can tops, or checkers for tokens.
- **Has to go potty *again.*** Go back to nighttime diapers for a while.
- **Hungry on a regular basis.** If really hungry, regularly include a small, simple snack before brushing teeth.
- **Is clearly frightened.** See p. 29.
- **Climbs out of bed.** Ignore this. Dress in warm pajamas if the floor is cold—or cover child later with a blanket. It's unlikely to last more than a few weeks. If a toddler climbs out of a crib, put the mattress on the floor for safety and childproof the room.
- **Won't stay in bedroom.** See p. 20.

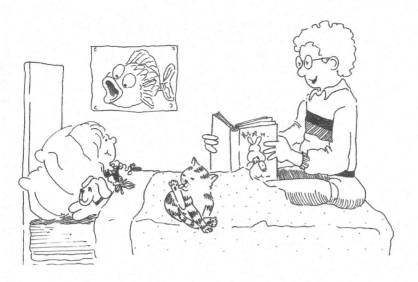

After bedtime books together, Emma used to settle quickly to sleep. Now 2½, she pleads for water, snacks, kisses, hugs, more stories, and to pee in the toilet. Mom set up a token system. After story time, Emma could exchange her two checkers for two requests. If, after spending her two tokens, Emma said she needed to go pee, Mom put her in a diaper despite the screaming and kicking. Realizing the limit was firm, Emma cried and fussed for 20 minutes for the next four nights, but then accepted the new token system.

The goal is to find your child's sleep window. Well-rested children generally fall asleep more easily than those who are over-tired. On the other hand, spending bored, restless time in bed while wide awake is rarely helpful. Sometimes kids stay up too late waiting for a parent to get home from work. Once they are age 2 or 3, have the absent parent call for a brief chat before bedtime.

Minds, Bodies, and Biorhythms

Not tired at bedtime. This commonly means that naptime is too long or too late. If your childcare program won't cooperate with a different nap routine, look for another program if possible. Sometimes, the entire day's schedule may need to shift earlier. See p. 27. A few children are "short sleepers" who need less sleep than we wish. They wake on their own in the morning and are in good spirits all day and evening. To get evening downtime for parents, set a time for kids to go to their rooms, and allow them to do quiet activities until they are tired.

Waiting for sleep to come. Some children routinely need 15-30 minutes to drift into sleep. Move bedtime earlier to allow for this time. Offer quiet music or soothing activities. Some high-energy children are tired, but can't lie still long enough for sleep to come. Encourage them to move *slowly*. For example, they can slowly stretch each hand, then foot, toward a corner of the bed. They can also do slow yoga stretches or hold different muscles tight and then relax them. To help preschoolers to think of relaxing, repetitive things to do, see p. 30.

Tired then wired at bedtime. Some children resist sleep because they don't want to miss what's going on. Others get tired, then revved up and wired. Such children find it stressful to be tired, and their bodies respond by pumping adrenalin into the bloodstream. This natural chemical, like coffee, can cause the jitters and can make sleep impossible. It's essential to understand this tired/wired pattern. By the time these children *look tired,* they may already be pumping adrenaline and be past their sleep window. They generally need to go down for sleep just *before* they start yawning and rubbing their eyes.

To predict, ask yourself, "How long has he been up?" "How tiring has her day been?" Their sleep window may look like a slight slowing down, a pause in activity, a calmer moment, or a glazed look. Get them ready for bed early, then put them in bed during the calm before the storm.

Exercise. Most children, especially high-energy ones, sleep better after lots of exercise during the day. Some children run wildly until bedtime then, when put in bed, fall dead asleep in a flash. Others have trouble falling asleep right after exercise. Some need 30 minutes and others two hours to settle for sleep after exercise. Adjust exercise accordingly.

Bath time. For many children a bath is relaxing. For others it's stimulating, in which case move their bath before dinner or to the morning.

Trouble after the weekend. Some children who stay up late on the weekend are then fussy and over-tired during the week. They may need two to five days to recover. Life is much easier if you stick to their regular schedule.

Night owl or morning lark. Genetics determine this tendency to wake early or stay up late. Such tendencies may not be a problem, or you may need to constantly nudge toward a schedule that works better in your family. See p. 27.

Effects of Light.
Most homes around the world are dimly lit compared to ours, which makes sleep come more easily. Bright lights and video screens (which beam light directly into the eyes) can delay sleepiness, especially in some people. Room lighting of 15 watts fluorescent (100 watts traditional) and even short bursts of bright light can delay sleep onset. If needed, dim room lights for 30-60 minutes before bedtime and use dark window coverings in summer. Avoid screen time for two hours before bedtime and no TV, video, or computer in the child's bedroom.

Irregular body rhythms. Most people have regular biological rhythms. Parents then know when kids will get tired and can set a routine that fits. For some children, when they get tired or how much sleep they need varies more than an hour from one day to the next—according to exercise, emotional tension, and other invisible factors. You may be able to nudge such irregular sleepers toward a more regular schedule. See p. 27. If you need regularity in your own life, set bedtime and provide quiet (unexciting) activities in the child's room while she waits for sleep.

For unknown reasons, our biologic clock counts closer to 25 hours per day rather than 24. This means a tendency toward gradually getting tired later and waking later. This 25-hour clock is stronger in some people than others. In such cases, carefully manage the child's daily schedule to better match our 24-hour days. See p. 27.

Fear of falling. A few people, upon closing their eyes, feel like they are falling. They don't know where their bodies are in space because they don't get strong clear messages from position sensors in their joints. Needless to say, this can make going to sleep very difficult. Try very specific positions such as head pressed against the top of the bed, or back against a wall, or hands pressed under a heavy mat. If preschoolers have trouble going to sleep, ask, "How do you feel when you close your eyes?"

Fear of the dark. Use a night light, or the doorway open to a lighted hall. Also see p. 29.

Food and drink. Sodas with caffeine easily keep children awake. Certain food dyes and additives affect energy and sleep in a small number of children. See *www.feingold.org*.

Medications. A few medicines make sleep more difficult. This includes many common treatments for asthma. Talk with your doctor about dose, timing, or about alternative medications. Use Tylenol® when needed for nighttime comfort with teething. Over-the-counter sleep medications, such as Benadryl® and melatonin, may help re-establish regular sleep after travel or illness. They should generally not be used on a regular basis. Be aware that some children have the opposite reaction to Benadryl®. It hypes them up instead of slowing them down.

Sleep Cues

Sleep cues are the physical signs and sensations we all use to feel safe and able to relax into sleep. Adults use body position, the familiar pillow, or warm body nearby, as well as the semiconscious awareness of our usual surroundings. Children also rely on familiar cues to relax into sleep.

Parent as sleep cue. Infants naturally use breast (or bottle), rocking, and contact with parents as their primary cue at bedtime *and during the night.* These patterns can continue happily for months or years. Whether it's nursing, stroking Mom's hair, or Dad's calm presence, when these sleep cues are more of a problem than a pleasure, it's time for a change. Some toddlers and preschoolers stay awake longer and longer to be sure that parents are still nearby. Others get upset during the night because their sleep cue snuck away.

Thumb or pacifier. Sucking can be an important way to relax into sleep, especially for high-energy kids. Current American culture pushes youngsters to grow up fast, so pacifiers are often discouraged early on. However, before age 3, sucking is one of the most reliable self-soothing tools available. For kids who are intense and find transitions hard, sucking can be helpful even longer. Pacifiers can be restricted to bed only so they don't limit daytime talking.

Dentists say that sucking thumb or a pacifier is not a problem before turning 3. Even if the shape of the jaw changes slightly due to long, strong sucking, the jaw returns to normal if preschoolers suck less after age 3. If your child is 3 and you are still concerned, check with your dentist to see whether continued sucking is a problem.

Bottle. As with thumbs and pacifiers, bottles are important to some children, especially before 3. If a bottle is your child's sleep cue, gradually dilute it more and more until it contains only water. Then tooth decay is not an issue. For some youngsters, drinking even water while lying down causes more ear infections. If that's the case, switch to a different sleep cue.

15

Blankets and bears. Little ones are most likely to get attached to a security object between 12 and 18 months. These items are helpful because they are reminders of parents. To encourage this connection, include the security object as part of nursing and bedtime rituals. Try knotting up one of Mom's tee shirts because it has her smell. **Textures** may also be important. For flexibility use a set of identical wash cloths or cut a favorite blanket into several parts.

Quiet. For sensitive children with very acute hearing, even small noises can be a problem. Use soft music, a fan, or a white noise machine that blocks other sounds.

How to Change Sleep Cues

Inborn temperament and age strongly affect the ease or difficulty of changing sleep cues. Some children adjust quickly and easily to increasing bedtime separation. Those who are highly sensitive, easily frustrated, or have difficulty with new things and transitions are likely to protest. For some, making changes in gradual steps results in a smooth transition. For others, resistance, fussiness, or outright screaming is inevitable. It's our job as parents to do what is best for the whole family, and it's the child's job to protest what is hard for him or her. Once the transition is complete, these kids will likely become as attached to the new system as the old.

Steps for changing sleep cues:
- **When**. Start new sleep cues at bedtime. Within one to two weeks many youngsters start using the new cues to get themselves back to sleep during the night. Consider stage of development, etc. See p. 7–8.
- **How many changes at a time.** Some youngsters do better with single, small changes. For example, stop rocking them to sleep but stay nearby while they adjust. Others get more angry because you are nearby yet won't pick them up. In that case, it's better to put them down and leave the room.
- **Where.** Teach new sleep cues in whatever bed you want the child to end up in. Becoming familiar with this new place is part of learning sleep cues.

- **Make new cues available.**
  Include the new teddy bear at story time. Put several pacifiers in the crib, or clip one to the mattress.

If nursing is the sleep cue, stop nursing at bedtime while your toddler is drowsy but still awake. Nurse a little earlier to avoid the child falling asleep at the breast. If you are together in a family bed you may need to sleep elsewhere for several days or weeks. *Expect fussing and crying.* See p. 21.

Progressive Waiting. This chart of "progressive waiting time" shows how long to wait before responding to crying. If the times seem too long, set shorter ones that feel right and you can stick to. When time is up, go in, say a few words, and leave, even though crying continues or gets louder. If crying is easing off, don't go in—you'll interrupt self-soothing. Most youngsters will be angry, not frightened. If genuine fear is an issue, see p. 29.

Feeling guilty?
Think how often loving adults give children what's needed and wanted. Toddlers and preschoolers build trust on the fact that adults *usually* respond positively. Of the 168 hours in a week, how many is your child content, and how many crying? There is no evidence that crying while learning new sleep cues causes psychological damage to toddlers and preschoolers who are well loved and cared for.

How Many Minutes to Wait			
Night #	1st wait	2nd wait	3rd and all additional waits
1	3	5	10
2	5	10	12
3	10	12	15
4	12	15	17
5	15	17	20
6	17	20	25
7	20	25	30

Based on Solve Your Child's Sleep Problems *by Richard Ferber, M.D., p 74*

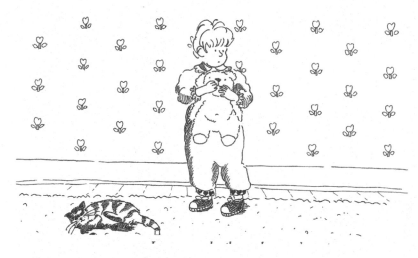

How long will it take? It depends on the child's age and temperament. Some parents are amazed that a few minutes of fussing for a night or two changes everything. On the other hand, intense 14-month-olds may scream for 45 minutes (just as they do because you take away the TV remote). If toddlers cry for more than an hour for more than three or four nights, they probably aren't ready to make this change. Some emotionally intense youngsters cry so hard that they vomit when upset. If you are confident that your plan is best for the family, go in, change the bedding, and continue from there.

Mom (or Dad or the sitter) stayed with Emma while she fell asleep—usually 15 minutes. But at 2½ Emma started staying awake longer and longer. Mom was sure Emma stayed awake to be sure she wasn't alone. When Mom was firm and left, Emma screamed. Dad said Emma needed new sleep cues. Mom was hesitant, but agreed. For a week they made Teddy a regular part of story time. The first two nights of progressive waiting, Emma screamed for 45 minutes. The next three nights she cried for 20 minutes, and the next four nights for 10. On the 9th night, she hugged her teddy, and didn't cry at all.

CHAPTER 5. Where Kids Sleep: How to Change It

There is no single right place for sleep. Traditionally, human babies slept next to their mothers for at least two years, when the next baby usually arrived. They then moved to the outer edge of the sleeping mat or bedded down with siblings or other relatives. Now, with smaller families and larger homes we have other options. Some children sleep in the family bed, others in their own rooms. Some fall asleep in the living room and are later carried to bed, while others remain in the living room because there is no other space. Some sleep in different places during the night.

As far as bed options, toddlers and preschoolers may sleep in the family bed, a toddler bed, a regular bed, or with a mat or sleeping bag on the floor. Parents may sleep in their own bed or in an extra bed in the child's room, or—during transitions—on sofa pillows or a mattress on the child's floor. Some parents, especially light sleepers, sometimes catch a good night's sleep *alone* on the living room sofa. (Do not sleep on a sofa with a baby or young child because of risk of suffocation to the child.)

Some parents enjoy the connection of nearby sleeping (or don't have another room) so are in no hurry to make changes. Others want a break from ongoing childcare or look forward to a more spontaneous nightlife of their own. The goal is to maximize sleep for the whole family, maintain an overall loving relationship with the child, as well as provide some downtime for parents.

If you hope for a bed without kids before they turn 3, it's often easier to shift before 2, when emotions often run stronger. If the change is because a new baby is coming, do so several months ahead of time to lessen feelings of jealousy.

Moving out of the crib. This is usually easy, especially if kids are told a few days ahead or even help choose or bring in the new bed. Children who are 35 inches tall may try to climb out of a crib and fall. Put the crib mattress on the floor or move child to a toddler bed. Childproof the room.

Moving to (and staying in) a separate room. A familiar place is important for sleep, as are relationships. Play together in the new room during the day and hold bedtime rituals there. Our presence helps this room become comfortable. From the family bed, there are two changes ahead. One is sleep without physical contact with parents and the other is sleep in a separate room. Sometimes it's easier to shift in two steps—separately in the same room and then to different rooms. As with other changes, children who are more sensitive, intense, easily frustrated, or have difficulty with transitions are likely to protest more or need more transition time. Parents may stay nearby (reading, resting, doing Yoga, etc.) while these children fall asleep in the new room. Some parents spend a few days or a couple of weeks sleeping on sofa pillows or a mattress in the child's room during the transition.

Reward children for staying in their room. Offer stars or give tokens to exchange for a treat when so many are earned. Say, "If you stay in your room, I can leave the door open."

Provide a *consequence* if they come out by walking them back consistently, with no eye contact and few words. Be more persistent than they are. Use a gate at the door or a childproof door handle cover on the inside door.

Hold the door closed for a short period if the child won't stay in the bedroom (start with 15 seconds and work up to 5-15 minutes by the sixth night). From outside the door, say nothing or calmly say, "It's bedtime." Avoid conversation. When time is up, open the door, say, "It's time to stay in your room and sleep." If the child leaves the room again, walk him back, close door, and continue holding and waiting according to plan. Most children will stay in their room by the third or fourth night. A few require more than seven days.

For Kim, in a studio apartment, separate rooms weren't an option. However, because Bryon kicked and thrashed while asleep, she needed him in a separate bed. She got a mattress that leaned against the wall during the day. Her first step was to snuggle next to Bryon as he went to sleep on his new mattress. After a week, she read nearby as he went to sleep. Whenever he climbed into her bed during the night, she returned him to his mattress. After two weeks, Bryon stayed on his mattress and Kim was finally sleeping well and waking up rested.

CHAPTER **6. Night Waking**

Most American parents assume *they* will be sleeping through the night by their baby's first birthday if not long before. Many are, and many are not. To change nighttime waking consider the causes.

How Common Is Night Waking?	
Age	**% of children who wake parents at night**
1 to 3 yr.	**About 30%.** Of these, 1/3rd wake parents several times per night, 1/3rd once per night, and 1/3rd once or twice per week.
3 yr.	**25%** wake parents 3 times per week.
4 yr.	**A few** wake parents occasionally because of nightmares.

Based on Is This a Phase? Child Development and Family Strategies, Birth to Age 6 *by Helen F. Neville*

Nighttime hunger. After 12 months (and generally much sooner), healthy youngsters don't *need* calories during the night. Nursing, however, may still be an important cue to relax back to sleep. If your child does seem genuinely hungry during the night, gradually cut the size of night feedings (nurse for shorter periods or put less in the bottle). Over the course of one to two weeks, with fewer calories at night, little ones automatically start eating and drinking more during the day. Once they are no longer really hungry at night, you can move on to other issues. Sharing the family bed, Mom would wake to find Beatriz was already nursing. Mom started wearing a tee shirt and belt to bed, announcing, "Boobies have gone night-night."

Trouble getting back to sleep. Children usually wake parents during the night because they haven't yet learned to get themselves back to sleep. See p. 15. Night waking is also more common before or during new phases of development. Highly sensitive youngsters may be more aware of and often more bothered by light, noise, or other slight changes during the night. Such interruptions may startle them awake and they therefore have trouble getting back to sleep. Cover windows with dark blinds if passing cars change room lighting. Also see p. 13. and 16.

Too hot or cold. Don't overdress sleeping children. If active youngsters roll out from under blankets, use warmer pajamas as needed. Sudden heat waves are likely to interrupt sleep, but over time most children get accustomed to warm nights.

Too much daytime sleep. Children only need a certain number of hours of sleep out of every 24. It may be less than you wish. If naps are too long or bedtime too early, your child may be awake during the night. See p. 27 and 28.

Illness. Fevers, teething, itchy skin, and earaches can interrupt nighttime sleep. Fluid in the ears can be more painful at night due to added pressure against the eardrum when lying down. Check with your doctor. Expect setbacks in night waking after illness.

Snoring. Whether or not children visibly wake up, snoring interrupts sleep and can cause fussiness the next day. Occasional snoring with colds and congestion is normal. However, allergies, large tonsils, and excess weight can cause ongoing, problematic snoring. Check with your doctor or nurse.

Gastro-Esophageal Reflux (GERD). If the muscle at the top of the stomach is weak, stomach acid may leak into the throat, especially if children are lying on their stomachs. This can cause painful burning in the throat. Acid may even reach the trachea (the airway), which sets off a cough/gag reflex to protect breathing. This reflex along with pain can startle the child awake, making it hard to fall back to sleep. Talk with your doctor or nurse.

The family bed had worked really well. Now, however, Mom wanted to stop nighttime nursing. Jesse, now 2, had a different opinion. Leah gradually cut night nursing shorter and shorter. Once Leah knew Jesse wasn't hungry during the night, she felt ready to take a stronger stand on teaching Jesse a new way to get back to sleep.

CHAPTER **7. Naps**

Naps are essential for young children's well-being and positive mood. We have little influence on *how much* sleep children need, but more influence on *when* they get it.

Naps: How They Change Over Time	
Age	**Naps**
12-21 mo.	Most drop morning naps.
3 yr.	90% still need afternoon naps.
4 yr.	50% still need afternoon naps.
5 yr.	25% still need afternoon naps.
6 yr.	Most don't nap in the afternoon unless it's the custom of the whole family.

Based on Healthy Sleep Habits, Happy Child *by Marc Weissbluth, M.D.*

Dropping naps. Youngsters usually start by skipping naps occasionally, then more often. It may be a rocky few weeks (or few months) until they shift completely. Once they drop a nap, total sleep need may be the same or less.

Sometime between 2 and 6 years, there is a biological shift in body hormones that allows children to stay in good spirits without an afternoon nap. If children still need a nap as they approach age 5, look for a morning kindergarten so they can nap in the afternoon.

Naps are too long. Long afternoon naps may make bedtime too late. We often hesitate to wake youngsters during an afternoon nap because they are fussy when woken. Waking at a different time in the cycle (light, deep, then light sleep) affects how easily they wake. Try waking them 15 or 30 minutes earlier or later.

Naps are too late. See p. 27.

Learning new sleep cues. Crying is common during this learning period. If your child cries for 30 minutes, get them up. Skip the nap and let them catch up on sleep later. Otherwise, they are likely to nap late and long, such that bedtime will be delayed and difficult.

Child gives up naps before parent is ready. Parents often rely on children's naps to catch up on work or sleep. Once naps are no longer needed, you can still enforce a quiet time: set up the bedroom with books, toys, or even an exercise ball for active kids to bounce on. Depending on the child, 20 minutes to an hour may be realistic. For a visual timer that even young children can understand, see *www.timetimer.com.*

Weekdays vs. weekends. Some children nap readily in childcare but not at home on weekends. You can simply accept this as the compliment it is—time with you is important. Or set up a rest time, as above. If children are short of sleep and fussy on the weekend, insist on a rest time which will hopefully turn into a nap.

Beatriz, 30 months, started skipping weekend naps. She napped easily at child care. Mom worried that Beatriz wasn't getting enough sleep. But Beatriz was generally in good spirits even in the late afternoon and evening. Apparently she was getting enough sleep. Because her parents were away long hours during the week, they enjoyed the extra time with Beatriz. However, they now had less time to connect as a couple. Rather than fight about naps, they set up a trade with another family to get some couple time every other Friday evening.

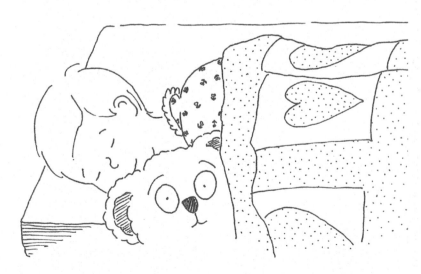

CHAPTER 8. Morning Issues

Like animals, we have a biological alarm clock loosely tied to daylight on our planet. Thus many children wake about the same time each morning *no matter when they went to sleep.* If they stayed up late last night, they still wake at their normal time, even though they didn't get a full night's sleep. They'll likely be fussy as a result. (A few kids sleep in late if they go to sleep late.) This set biological alarm clock means that many children will wake at their normal time even if we put them to bed earlier than usual.

Wakes too early. Dark curtains may help by cutting morning light. Moving the entire sleep schedule later may work. See p. 28.

Wakes too late. If we wake children up in the morning, they start each day sleep deprived and are often fussy. To move bedtime earlier, see p. 27. Some parents need to take children to childcare very early in order to get to work. If so, try to maximize sleep. Put youngsters to bed in next day's clothes or take them to day care in their pajamas. Pack a breakfast for them to eat when they wake.

Wakes up fussy. Some children may wake up fussy or crying and remain grouchy or somber until they fully wake. Greet these kids with a glass of milk, juice, or a snack in bed. Then they get needed calories on board before getting up and have time to wake gradually. Lay out clothes the night before to avoid early morning decisions or surprises.

Wakes early on Saturday. Just as adults may wake early due to excitement, some children wake *early* on Saturday in order to watch cartoons. This is a problem if they are tired and fussy later in the day. Unplug or remove the TV.

Extra weekend sleep for parents. Once children are 3, we may be able to get some extra sleep by leaving a snack and something interesting by the bedside. As needed for safety, put a gate at the child's door or at the door to the kitchen. Many 4s can entertain themselves for a while in the morning.

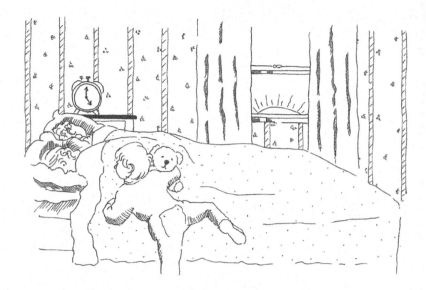

As a baby, Terrell woke up crying every morning. Now 3, he's grumpy and uncooperative. Mom suddenly realized that she's always in a better mood after morning coffee. So instead of nagging Terrell to get up and get dressed, she took a glass of milk to his room. When she returned in 15 minutes, he was in a much better mood and ready to get up.

CHAPTER 9. Sleep Schedules: How to Change Them

Though we can't change how much sleep our children need, we can influence when they get it. If children wake too early for our comfort, a later schedule may work better. If they stay up too late or we have to wake them in the morning, then an earlier schedule may work better. The chart below tells how to change sleep schedules. This process can also help shift children's schedules when clocks change in the spring and fall.

Move schedule earlier. If your child goes to sleep too late or wakes up too late, try following the chart below.

Changing Schedule by Waking Child Earlier	
Amount to change	**15 min.** every day or two until you reach the desired schedule.
When to start	Start by **waking the child earlier** in the morning.
Morning light	Lots of morning light. (Sunlight if possible)
Wake-up time	Wake children up at first. With time they'll usually start waking earlier on their own.
Eating times	Start 15 min. earlier to match morning waking.
Exercise	Encourage exercise in the morning and mid afternoon. Try to avoid vigorous exercise in the evening.
Naps	Start 15 min. earlier. Avoid naps that are too late or too long. (No more than 90 min. to 2 hrs.) Wake children if needed.
Evening light	No video or computer time after dinner because light delays sleepiness. Lower room light 30-60 min. before bedtime. Use dark window covers if needed.
Bedtime	At first, children may not be sleepy at the new bedtime. If so, let them stay up until their usual one. Once the new morning wake-up time is easy, then move bedtime earlier. For children who get wired when over-tired, it may be better to start both wake-up and bedtime 15 min. earlier.
Use the yearly time change	In the fall, clock time "falls back" an hour. Kids automatically wake an hour earlier.

Move schedule later. If your child wakes too early or goes to sleep too early, try following the chart on page 28.

27

Changing Schedule by Waking Child Later	
Amount to change	**15 min.** every day or two until you reach the desired schedule.
When to start	Start by **keeping the child up later** in the evening.
Morning light	Use dark window covers if needed.
Wake-up time	It may be a few days before children to start sleeping later in the morning.
Eating times	Start 15 min. later to match bedtime.
Exercise	Moderate exercise in the afternoon and evening—but avoid getting over-tired.
Naps	Start 15 min. later.
Evening light	Lots of light (especially sunlight) in the afternoon and early evening.
Bedtime	Keep the child up 15 min. later each night or two until reaching the new schedule.
Use the yearly time change	In the spring, clocks "spring forward" an hour. Kids automatically go to bed an hour later.

Kim woke Bryon for daycare each morning before work. She realized it would be better for him to start his days fully rested, so she changed his sleep schedule. Each weekend, while she was home with him, she moved his entire schedule 15 minutes earlier—waking time, meals, light, and exercise. After four weeks, he was going to bed an hour earlier, and waking on his own in the morning.

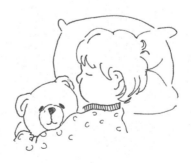

Like frightened adults, frightened children find it hard to relax into sleep. Fear and worry are somewhat more common in youngsters who are emotionally intense and cautious in new situations. Little ones often react to our upsets about finances, illness, partner problems, or work. Sometimes, leaving children alone at night reminds us of painful separations from our own past. Clarify in your own mind who is under stress. Identify children's fears and find ways to calm them.

Imaginary fears. A preschooler's growing imagination makes it hard for her to separate fantasy from reality. For 2s and especially 3s, any dark corner can easily transform into a scary creature. Fight fantasy with fantasy. Point out with confidence that "Teddy Bear will chase scary creatures out of the room." Supply a magic wand, a flashlight, or a spray bottle of magic water that smells "yucky" to monsters and makes them leave.

Nightmares. Nightmares commonly start around 2½ years. They are a challenge before children can talk. At 2, Beatriz repeatedly woke at night, crying with fear. One morning Mom gave her paper and crayons to scribble a picture of the bad dream. Mom and Beatriz put the paper in the garbage can with a brick on top until the garbage truck came and took it away. Beatriz's bad dreams stopped.

Preschoolers commonly have nightmares about dogs, monsters, and occasionally ghosts. Nightmares often relate to fear from earlier that day—scary videos, or a big dog (or angry parent) that barked. These strong, leftover feelings come back at night dressed in different costumes.

Starting at 3 or 4, have children tell their dream in the morning then add a new and better ending. "What would be a *good* ending to this dream?" "Tell me again; I like that ending!" Byron complained of a nighttime ghost. Mom asked, "What do you think it wants to say?" and "What will make it feel better so it won't bother you?" This process helps children feel more control over their worries. Some children sleep better after asking for "good dreams" at bedtime, or saying a prayer for a peaceful night's sleep.

Helpful Views. If the room is very dark, use a nightlight so children know where they are when they awake. Post a picture of Mom or Dad beside the bed to remind toddlers and 3s that you are nearby.

Worry. With 4s and 5s, review the day's events. "What was hard today?" "What might make that easier next time?" End on a positive note: "What's something that went well today?" Even as young as 3, some kids lie awake wondering about the next day. Review tomorrow's plans at bedtime. If children are still worried, put a "worry envelope" by the bedside. Write down their worries and put it in the envelope: "This worry will stay here in the envelope so it won't bother you tonight." Tell preschoolers that people often wake up in the morning with answers for their worries.

Fours and 5s can use mental pictures to manage worry. Say, "You have a TV in your head with three channels. Channel 1 is the worry channel. It shows things we worry about. Channel 2 is the answer channel. It shows ways to make things better. Channel 3 is the relaxing channel. There, you can blow up balloons of different colors, pet a cat, ride a bike, or rock on an air mattress in a pool of water. The relaxing channel is the best one to look at while you're waiting for sleep."

Family stress. Tell children when they are *not* the cause of our worry. Tell them we will find solutions to adult problems. Children commonly have nightmares after major stress such as natural disasters. At such times, they usually sleep better near familiar adults. Listen to their concerns during the day. If signs of stress are severe or continue for more than a month, get help from doctors, counselors, or social service agencies.

Night terrors are different from nightmares. They usually occur early in the night (1-3 hours after bedtime) during periods of very deep sleep. With night terrors, children don't recognize us even if their eyes are open. They are most common when children are stressed or tired, such as when they have just dropped a nap. Stay nearby but don't try to wake them. If night terrors occur several nights in a row, wake the child just *before* they usually happen. If they continue, check with your doctor.

Sleepwalking is most common between 3 and 8 years. Until they outgrow it, protect young ones with a baby gate at the bedroom door, the kitchen door, or a high secure lock on front and back doors. Sleepwalking may be more common when children are over-tired or under stress.

Terrell woke with nightmares about monsters. He became afraid of his bed where the monsters appeared. Mom realized she'd been short tempered with Terrell recently, due to stress at work. Mom said, "Do you remember when I shouted last night because you were pulling the dog's tail? A dream is about you yourself, pretending to be different. I think that in your dream you were scared, just like when I yelled at you. And in your dream I looked like a scary monster. I'm sorry I yelled at you. I love you." Terrell's nightmares stopped.

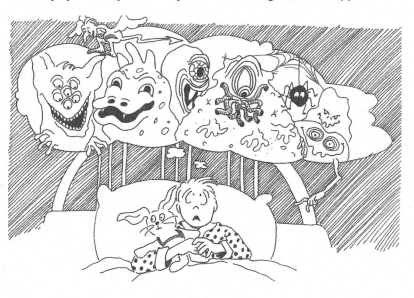

Are Things Better?

I hope you can now see some light at the end of the tunnel. Be patient as change usually takes time. Because change takes work, too, things often get harder before they get easier. If you're still feeling really stuck, refer to chapter 2, "Keys to Sleep Success" and take stock. Who is having difficulty? Is your goal realistic? Is this a good time for change? Have you overlooked anything?

Congratulate yourself if you have solved your family's sleep problems—at least until your child grows into a new stage. Keep this guide at hand for your children's futures and pass it on to another tired parent when you no longer need it.

Best wishes for a good night's rest!

Bibliography

Ferber, Richard, M.D. *Solve Your Baby's Sleep Problems.* New York: Simon & Schuster, 1985, 2006

Huntley, Rebecca. *The Sleep Book for Tired Parents: Help for Solving Children's Sleep Problems.* Seattle: Parenting Press, 1991

Neville, Helen F., B.S., R.N. *Is This a Phase? Child Development and Parent Strategies, Birth to Age 6.* Seattle: Parenting Press, 2007

Sears, William, M.D. *The Baby Sleep Book.* New York: Little, Brown and Company, 2005

Weissbluth, Marc, M.D. *Healthy Sleep Habits, Happy Child.* New York: Ballantine Books, 2004